LOOKING IN THE MIRROR

LOOKING IN THE MIRROR

A POWERFUL BOOK RELATIG TO LIVING WITH BELL'S PALSY

Kay K. Balgemann

ISBN: 1516951743
ISBN 13: 9781516951741

PREFACE

THIS BOOK STARTED out to be a journal of the events taking place on my journey with Bells Palsy. My intentions were to document it for a couple of months. The original medical diagnosis in the hospital indicated I could expect a 2 to 4 month recovery from Bell's Palsy.

My primary health care doctor suggested I consider having surgery on the left side of my face in order to loosen the nerves. I chose not to have the surgery. The suggested medical procedure had not been proven effective and I feared that something might "go wrong", permanently damaging my facial muscles. Months went by and I was still struggling with all the sensations.

So this is an accounting of the phases I have gone through, in hopes of helping others understand the disease and its effect on one's life. I've tried to help the reader understand the personal side of someone inflicted with a facial change and how you might support their need for acceptance and love.

I also wanted to share my own theory of how a determination to be the best you can be with whatever is put in your way; how to appreciate other's plight and move toward them and not away from them, shutting them off from those experiences you take for granted.

I hope, after reading this, and if you are suffering from Bell's Palsy, you will understand that there is hope for you to regain your self-worth and how you will and can still take hold of your life and be more than you think you can be! If you are reading this out of curiosity, that you might come away with a greater understanding of the disease and be more aware of those around you who have encountered disabilities of any kind.

It is my sincere desire that after reading this book, you will find hope knowing that anyone stricken with Bell's Palsy can achieve self-worth and regain a quality of life greater than ever expected.

DISCLAIMER

THE AUTHOR NOR publisher shall not have any liability to anyone with respect to any damage or loss caused by any instructions contained in this book or by products or services recommended.

TABLE OF CONTENTS

CHAPTER 1

INTRODUCTION

As I AM writing this, thoughts come into my mind which I have had regarding this whole episode of my life. Questions arise as to why I have experienced life this way and how anyone could ever expect to get through a time of such an immense, radical trial without questioning one's very existence.

So, in a time of deep consideration, I have decided to explore all the avenues I can to help explain what has happened in my life, in order to show someone else the avenue they might choose in their own experiences with a disease called Bell's Palsy.

It is to be understood that this has not been the only *bump* in my life's journey so far. All of us experience tidal waves of unexpected mishaps that we either allow to *define us* in the eyes of others or that we embrace and *conquer* through a belief that we are here for a purpose and are gifted as individuals to withstand what has been given to us.

These reflections are offered as a help to understanding why I've chosen to write so openly about the scary world of having an extended version of Bell's Palsy... a condition that really tests your strength as a human being, a condition that makes you look beyond what you once thought was important ... and look deep into your soul's eye to understand what God is intending you to be.

My tomorrows will never be like my yesterdays … but the experience of dealing with this every day and every waking hour shall make my tomorrows a grateful existence. There is joy if you can manage to look beyond yourself and not rely on how you had dreams and visions of grandeur. Those were yesteryear's thoughts, but today one's mind must accept reality thoughts and how you must navigate your everyday life, not pondering on the whys of yesterday, but use your reality to bring hope to help others by means of your affliction.

How many people do we know who deal with afflictions on a daily basis, but whom we never consider who they really are? The person who lives alone because of certain circumstances in their lives, no one is with them as they struggle with a disease or handicap; the person who is in a special facility living a life they would never have planned for themselves; the child who is afflicted with a crippling disease, keeping their spirits up by slowly making small daily progress—all these folks are reminders of just how much we have to be thankful for, no matter what our circumstances.

CHAPTER 2

EUGENE A VISION OF FUTURE EVENTS

Today I'm remembering Eugene, a young man whom I met when I was 13 or 14 years old, and the thoughts that went through my mind back then suddenly come back to my memory as though it was yesterday. Growing up in Lancaster, Ohio, I had a really best friend Mary, who lived next door. She was older than I, we played together and talked across the "what Chicago folks would call" *gangway* between our houses, between our bedroom windows. One day she asked if I would like to go with her family to visit her cousin Eugene...and I agreed. It was a Sunday, and I joined Mary, her older sister Madeline and her parents, all piling into their family car and drove through town till we came to Eugene's house. Eugene's mom answered the door and graciously led the way past the modest living room to what was meant to be a dining room, but now had a hospital bed, dresser and other chairs for visitors. Eugene was in the bed, and he looked at us and smiled, waving his hand in such an awkward manner, that I instantly realized he was afflicted with something I had never encountered before. His mom explained to me, in a very matter-of-fact manner that Eugene was born with Cerebral Palsy. The doctors had suggested that he be placed in a facility with others like him … but she chose to raise him and take care of his needs at home.

HE SPOKE IN an awkward way, the only way his muscles would allow, and it required his mom to sometimes interpret what he was trying to say. It was such a difficult- thing to see and I often think that perhaps that experience was provided to help me later in my own future life experiences.

And as it turned out, I gave birth to a son who was also afflicted with Cerebral Palsy. His story I will share at another writing.

CHAPTER 3

LIFE BEFORE BELL'S PALSY

THIS STORY IS about my recent health experiences and how my perception of being healthy has been altered. As long as looking in the mirror showed me a face which I had been told was attractive and which always appeared happy and carefree, life was good.

We will begin with the time before my health changed my entire outlook on the world around me.

The last 2–3 years have seen such trials, all lived out by relying on my faith and prayers. However, my earlier choices were not biblically driven, only selfishly driven ... as my quest for a successful life always seemed just another opportunity away. I know my God has forgiven me for my past sins in making unwise choices, both in my private life and public business life—but I am haunted by this tale of woes.

When Hank and I were first married, in June of 1998, I was about to close a family food business that had failed. Hank offered to help and we tried to do it together, my believing that it (the idea for a food business) had been a *gift from God*.... Now not knowing why things had happened in such a way, I was questioning my faith and God's purpose for my life. We continued to attend church and found relief in leaning on the encouraging Bible messages each week. Willow Creek Community Church of South Barrington, IL, became our rock, the only place God's peace seemed to find us and give us strength to continue. The founding minister, Bill Hybles, and the many gifted ministries of this church fed us the teachings that we most needed to hear to sustain us.

Four years ago, Hank and I were returning from church, talking about meeting with our friends with whom we were planning a picnic at a park up in Northern Illinois. All of a sudden that moment turned into a tragic scene, as we were involved in an auto collision, totaling our van and forever changing our lives. The injuries were minor, then, but the aftereffects were enormous. Hank's back has never been the same, to the point that our personal physical relationship has been compromised. However, with physical therapy and chiropractic adjustments, his back is improving.

We had just recovered from a bankruptcy and my personal emotional wellness seemed unsteady. Though I functioned, I had to deal with a deformed foot, requiring surgery, then a mini-stroke (transient ischemic attack –TIA), leaving me somewhat weak on my left side. Then, soon after that, I encountered two infections: one E. coli that was treatable in the hospital, another (from beef) for which we were told "there was no cure." I was told that my system should be able to take care of it in time, and if my system could not, I would die!

We left for Palm Springs the day after I was released from the hospital. Tickets had been purchased months in advance, however, we had had to cancel and rebook due to the accident. Once at the airport, I was wheeled in a wheel chair…not strong enough to endure the security lines and the walk to the departure gate.

Once in Palm Springs, we stayed with our neighbors who own a home there … the sunshine, laughter and change of scenery really was what the doctor ordered! I did recover from both E. coli's.

Life seemed to be somewhat normal for a period of time.

CHAPTER 4

THE MIRROR

OCTOBER, 2012

Then, the unforeseeable thing happened. I got up as usual. Went to the kitchen table to sit and plan my day as was my practice. My husband walked in our back door, started up the short stairway to the kitchen. He could look directly at me from the stairway's half-wall. Before I could say anything to him, he said in a startled voice, "Kay, go look at yourself in the mirror." Looking back on that very moment, I remember reaching up to my face with both hands as there was a tingling sensation for a brief second on the left side of my face. I hurriedly walked into our washroom and looked in the mirror. I squealed in horror. I had no idea at the time what was happening; it was frightening. My left eye was frozen open. Looking in the mirror, who had I become? It was a face I did not recognize and one I would not have chosen.

Nothing could have prepared me for what I saw. My left eye was wide open ... more so than I would have ever thought possible. I could not blink ... the rest of the left side of my face was frozen in place! I had recently had cataract surgery on both eyes and was enjoying good vision and now this!

Having Bell's Palsy reminded me of the biblical people Jesus knew who had leprosy. I often wondered how they felt and what would I have done if I were born into this world in their condition.

We learn very little about them in the Bible, other that they kept to themselves and wore clothing that covered the afflicted areas of their body. Even though I had not changed to that extent, the disease I have encountered, Bell's Palsy, has definitely made me feel different and even somewhat unacceptable. Unacceptable to whom? Not God certainly, for He loves me no matter what. Unacceptable to Hank, to the outside world … to those who don't know me other than the way I looked before?

There were many early mornings when I sought out a quiet spot in our home where I could weep till there were no more tears.

CHAPTER 5

THE DIAGNOSIS

THAT FIRST MORNING, Hank and I were both frightened. We immediately called our neurologist. Then hearing instructions to go directly to the hospital's emergency room seemed to confirm our greatest fear—that I must have had or was in the process of having a stroke. The drive to the hospital seemed endless, even though it was only ten minutes away. I remember praying and trying to keep back the tears…!

Standing in line in the emergency room, I reminded Hank that the doctor had said to force our way past those waiting in line ahead of us. Hank immediately got the attention of the staff by saying there was a possible stroke patient waiting, and then all things seemed to happen at once. I was now in a cubicle area, an IV magically in my left arm, and then a doctor was standing at the end of my bed saying "you're not having a stroke, but you do have a case of Bell's Palsy … and it will probably all be gone in a couple of months!" Swell, I thought, I should be good for the holidays, Thanksgiving and Christmas.

No such luck! Does this ever end, I remember thinking. Of all the obstacles, this really seemed the most devastating. Never thinking of myself as being vain, but now unable to look at myself in a mirror without cringing, I was afraid to face whatever was to be.

The doctors at the hospital had said that in a few months I would be as good as new, that this condition would surely go away on its own. However, Hank did research on the computer, and YouTube folks and other medical websites told us that that isn't always the case … that in some instances it never goes completely away.

CHAPTER 6

DEFINITION AND HOPE

To BETTER UNDERSTAND the definition of this disease in today's world, I went to the internet and learned that

"Bell's Palsy is a form of *__facial paralysis__* resulting from a dysfunction of the cranial nerve VII (the *__facial nerve__*) causing an inability to control facial muscles on the affected side.. Named after Scottish anatomist *__Charles Bell__*, who first described it, Bell's Palsy is the most common acute *__mononeuropathy__* (disease involving only one nerve) and is the most common cause of acute facial nerve paralysis (>80%).

Bell's Palsy is defined as an idiopathic unilateral facial nerve paralysis, us-ually self-limiting. The hallmark of this condition is a rapid onset of partial or complete paralysis that often occurs overnight. In rare cases (<1%), it can occur bilaterally resulting in total facial paralysis.[1] [2]

It is thought that an inflammatory condition leads to swelling of the facial nerve. The nerve travels through the skull in a narrow bone canal beneath the ear. Nerve swelling and compression in the narrow bone canal are thought to lead to nerve inhibition, damage or death."

A friend suggested I check into an alternative treatment by a doctor/ chiropractor physician who incorporates Kinesiology into his treatments. The treatments for me also included changing my diet and exercise. After learning what foods my body was really allergic to, this made me focus on things other than my appearance. My husband joined me in this quest for better body health by eating more greens, rice, eggs, vegetables and getting completely away from other dairy products. I began to feel more *in charge* and had feelings of *hope* at last.

CHAPTER 7

EXPERIENCES

I JUST TURNED 70 years old and on what should have been a great day for me to celebrate all the lives who have been part of my life, I chose to keep the celebration limited to include only the ones who are the closest to me. I just could not bring myself to consent to having a 70th Birthday Party.... We just went with our closest family members to a local pub and shared a meal. I felt every eye on me and only ate small portions, as controlling my chewing while drooling out of the left side of my mouth was very strange to me ... and I knew it must have been awkward for others to watch, even while I kept a napkin close to the drooling side of my mouth, as though I was covering it all up.

MARCH, 2013 –

We were in church that day sitting down front as usual ... me with my dark sunglasses as I had done since my facial appearance was changed by the Bell's Palsy. I had my left eye frozen open, and a tape covered my eyelid closed so the eye would not dry out.

Reverend Harvey Carey, from Detroit, Michigan, was the guest speaker that day. We approached him after the service to ask him to pray for my healing. He asked what else was going on in our lives, as I could not help tearing up as the overwhelming emotions seemed to release.

I could not respond, so Hank started telling a short version of our lives starting with the fact that in the last decade we had experienced a failed business, personal bankruptcy which we completed in 5 years; we were involved in an automobile collision that destroyed our van and left Hank with serious back problems and me with a foot injury. Then I had a TIA, 2 colon diseases (E. coli) at one time, no cure for one … doctors had said nothing they could do for me if my body could not fight it off, then Bell's Palsy. The speaker encouraged me to publish my story so that others may learn from my experiences.

I remember one Sunday, at church, waiting for the opening of the main entrance to the auditorium, when two women came up to me and wanted to pray for me right there on the spot! I felt loved and cared for by the Holy Spirit, and I know my ability to handle the next several months was directly due to this incident. From this moment on, I learned of many others who have had this affliction and, therefore, I knew I was not alone in this and that really helped in my mental outlook.

I recall folks who knew me now looking at me and I could tell they were wondering what was different about how I looked … once I said what was going on, they seemed relieved and were so supportive.

JULY, 2013 -

Today, July 26, 2013, I have improved with the help of a chiropractic physician, specializing in Kinesiology, focused on my nutritional choices and readjusting my body's frame and, for lack of the terminology I need here, the pressure points that control my mobility and attempt to lessen or reverse the osteoporosis that I've been dealing with as well. The doctor is a Christian and has a unique personality.

He is blessed with a keen sense of humor which he mixes in with his attempt to exhibit a relaxed (usually in the form of laughter) state while he jerks, manipulates and evaluates what he needs to do to correct/balance his patient's present needs. In my case, I feel completely rejuvenated when I leave his office. I stand erect, and walk without the feeling I might fall to the left, the muscles in my face respond to the lightness of conversation and the almost angel-like effect the whole experience is. I might add this angel has tilted wings, just because of the twinkle in his eyes when he has told of a funny experience and realizes he's accomplished his mission—while you have been focused on the story he's telling, he's maneuvered your body in a quick unexpected jolt—of which you immediately understand why the *funny story*. You not only feel relieved of discomfort but feel lighthearted as well. It is something that just can't be explained. I prefer to think that God has given this doctor certain *powers* that we may have only heard about in the Bible —such as healing by the human touch of Jesus or one of his disciples.

My face is almost back to normal, but my speech is impaired as the left side of my mouth refuses to move when I speak … making me slur at times. The look of frustration my friends give me … what can they do … how should they be able to make out what I say when this happens? Anyhow, it isn't the end of the world as I know it … but it has become a different one for me.

CHAPTER 8

LIFE CHANGES

AUGUST, 2013

It has been over a year now and I'm still treating my Bell's Palsy. I've become used to the mirror looking back at me. With the help of *shock treatment* devices made to shock the nerves back to doing their job (instead of being stiff in place) and exercises I've learned from videos of others who have suffered, I am now *better*, and perhaps the best I can be.

Besides focusing on the changes in my appearance, I've learned to focus on exercise and on a different way of eating. Vegetables and fruits are really important to me now, and the result of this change is that I've lost 20 lbs. and am much more mobile than I ever was.

I've learned that my body overreacts to flour, sweets and red meat … and in compensating for this, of course, my husband has had to change his eating habits! I was not going to cook two separate meals—one for him and one for me! He has learned to love cauliflower, smashed and seasoned like mashed potatoes … sandwiches without bread, sweet potatoes in more ways than I can count, fish this and fish that, turkey … and he does without gravies, baked goods and chocolate! This is living?

Seriously though, there are foods that one should not eat—as was stated by my chiropractic doctor—that are not good for you, whether you have Bell's Palsy or are merely looking to get healthy (via weight loss). Those foods to avoid are soy milk, artificial sugar, margarine and orange juice. Whole wheat breads are to be avoided as well, because they are full of fatty chemicals.

Easier said than done, when you've been eating differently your whole life. However, the end results are well worth it. Keeping one's focus on doing this is another thing. We are human, and falling off the wagon—e.g. eating a favorite dessert or a once-favorite whole wheat bread sandwich can trigger the slouchy, no energy and bloating feelings of our past.

Finding foods that satisfy my "new look" needs is simple today, with technology at my fingertips. You need only to find a web site such as Betternutrition.com where there are all kinds of suggested meals, snacks to choose from and to include in your daily diet. Good things to start including in your diet are avocado, chia seeds and ginger. And where oh where would you stick these in your diet? If you are like I was, avocados, chia seeds and ginger were never staples in our diet growing up ... so how do you eat them, and why should you eat these foods?

The first new item I started including in my diet was the avocado. I experimented with how I was going to use this ... and find I enjoy the flavor in a fresh salad and crumbled in an egg omelet with turkey bacon and onion. The reason I began including this is that it has been shown to lower cholesterol levels, and it seeks out pre-cancerous and cancerous oral cancer cells and destroys them.

The chia seeds are full of protein, calcium, fiber and omega-3 fatty acids, and they pack a huge punch for one's workout. Adding a tablespoon with a banana, frozen fruit, greens and almond milk in a blender makes a great smoothie to start my morning with. If I think of it, I will sprinkle on my yogurt snack during the afternoon.

Ginger, on the other hand, is an herb that I still need to try as it is proclaimed to do wonders in treating many disorders: coughs, digestive disorders, sore throats, etc. (See MyRecipes.com for more suggested recipes.)

We laugh because our home has become a workout center without a gym. Every morning both of us do our own set of exercises, stretches, and weather permitting walk outside, or stay indoors on the treadmill for 30 minutes. Hank looks and is healthier and slimmer than I've ever seen him—now my 73-year-old *hunk*. The benefit for my Bell's is that I am not focused on how my facial looks are, but more focused on a total wellness.

Every morning, I spend a few moments with my Heavenly Father and ask for His guidance, and with tears, I sometimes express my feeling of unworthiness as there are so many others suffering from much more in their lives.

When I'm at church now, folks are used to my appearance … and it seems to be getting better, but personally—the feeling from within, is not how it was. I mean the left side of my face still feels stiff as though there is a plaster coating on the outside of my skin. The only way I can tell how it really must look to others, is to look in a mirror and make what should be normal glances, stares, shifts of expression …

and really observe how my nerves react to my efforts. It is in this way I've taught myself how not to smile (if I smile the way **it used to feel normal to smile**, the left side of my face or mouth contorts or overreacts so that I have a *clown like* look). I can mindfully hold my right side somewhat in place when I smile, or talk, for that matter … and I find it is acceptable.

A quick ritual I do, when the nighttime comes, while taking off my liquid makeup, which I wear to cover what imperfections my skin now has, is that I avoid looking in any mirror before going to bed. To be so vain, what does this say about me? We believe that our looks (how others see us) is the most important thing and that our future successes depend on us looking **the** best. I can remember as a young girl comparing my appearance with those of the *in group...*

If I could talk to that young girl today, knowing the things I do, I might tell her that God loves her just the way he made her and that the reason she was thinking others "have it better with newer fashions and outgoing personalities" … these things mean nothing to her Heavenly Father. He has given her all she needs to live a life full of love and free choices.

As a high school student, I taught 3-4 year olds every Sunday at our local United Methodist Church, in Lancaster, Ohio. There were usually 10-12 children in that early service class. Always a particular boy came (I'll refer to him as Johnny), his hair combed, parted on one side, wearing his *Sunday shirt*, light slacks, white socks and dark shoes. Always with **wet** pants, as though he wet himself, or someone just didn't take time to change him before coming to church. Johnny knew that I would have a change for him, changing his underwear and socks which were always soaked. I'd rinse out his wet clothes, hang them over the small register in the bathroom … and by the time his mom came to get him, the warm underwear and socks were back on him, and he always gave me the biggest grin every time he left. Johnny never had much to say or contribute in class, because I'm sure he felt embarrassed knowing the other children knew what had happened. However, he listened intently to all the Bible stories that were read in class, and squeezed his eyes closed tight when we prayed together. Although he came from a different environment than most of the others, the other children did not make fun of him or tease him. It is said that children are not born with prejudice or hate, they have to be taught by adults to have those negative feelings. I was very proud of that class!

CHAPTER 9

A NEW SEASON - FALL

FALL CAME WITH the brisk air of what had been my favorite season of the year!

What could be more refreshing than the cool touch of that first awakening step out of the warm bed? Why now is it not that way anymore? The cold air hitting the affected left side of this new face I have just seems to stiffen the feeling, and merely making a smile, or even yawning, is a reminder that we must start all over again today … but more intensely, exercising the muscles, making them move and trying to do natural expressions in front of the mirror.

So now I've decided that I must give myself that extra hour or two in the early morning to be ready for my husband when he gets up and is ready for his day. Sitting at the table for breakfast, I will be able to tell by the way he gazes at me, whether I have fallen back in my recovery or if it is OK. How I long for those days when I felt at ease and knew he got only pleasure out of his looking at me in the morning.

People usually go through their days doing "what they need to do on their to-do list," and unless there is a physical element that they are dealing with that slows that process down, life is full and good. I never thought of others with difficulties as struggling or having issues that made their lives so uncomfortable. I guess I just figured, that was the way it was for them, and so what!

Well, I know better now. Other folks with afflictions have much more of a meaning to me now ... it is an uncomfortable way to live, and only through loving, caring folks, whether they be family members, neighbors, church friends or even strangers ... and the Almighty Heavenly Father, can that life be fulfilling!

CHAPTER 10

THE HUMOR FACTOR

RECENTLY I WAS at a conference for Christian women and was privileged to meet a lady who was struggling with her weight gain. We talked about similar issues, one of those being the fact that when walking down a hall or on a street, *some* (or we should say *many*) folks, would rather look down to the ground as they are passing you by, rather than look you in the eye and acknowledge your "hello." As she was once a beautiful woman, and I was considered nice looking, this insignificant ignorant gesture from folks, who just can't imagine why one has such physical challenges, is like being slapped in the face. The aftermath of those incidents leaves you with an uncomfortable feeling when walking into a crowded room, or being any part of any social event!

So I have found that humor changes the way I feel about myself ... and allows the other person to let down that guard of "How do I treat this person?" They can laugh and release that emotion that holds them back from having a relationship with me. I find myself praying so that I can present a loving image even though my physical self looks less than loving to someone's first glance.

When there is a lull in conversation with anyone who is seeing me for the first time in this new state, I like to relate a funny story. Folks will watch me tell it, knowing I'm enjoying this ... and then they have time to "adjust or get used to who I am now." It's about the time when

I was young and my uncle gave me two small ducklings. I named them "Donald & Daisy." We lived on a busy street in the center of town, an unlikely place to raise ducklings! Dad built them a cage in the backyard, but when I was outside they followed me around the neighborhood and it was not unusual to see my friends and I and the ducks sitting on our front porch having a great time!

Donald and Daisy were very loving, running their long necks around your neck if you picked them up and quacking in delight! Then Daisy was suddenly killed when the cage was accidently blown over and landed on her. I was devastated. My neighborhood friends helped in giving her a funeral in the backyard.

Dad decided Donald needed a new mate, so we took him to the local park. Dad pulled the car up to the big lake threw Donald as far as he could out in the middle of the lake where there were a lot of other ducks. We all thought Donald would really be pleased. I'll never forget him looking as though he was walking on top of the water, as he spread his wings, and yelled at us … flying, or walking back across the water to reach us. Dad threw him in again, then jumped back into the car and we left! Dad was sure Donald would just get together with the other ducks as soon as we were gone.

The next Sunday after church we went back to the lake … and no Donald! He wore a red identification tag on one leg … so we would know him. I got out of the car, started walking and at last I could hear his quack (I'd know his quack anywhere). There was a large shelter on the hill behind the lake, with a large family reunion going on that day. I could see Donald strolling around the edges of the shelter. I called his name, he turned toward me, and running, quacking and flapping his wings ... followed me to the car, I opened the door and he jumped in! He loved people, not other ducks!

Donald finally ended up on my grandpa's farm ... and spent the rest of his days following my grandpa around while he tended to his chores. Grandpa was a tall, distinguished-looking gentleman and he looked very out of place with a duck following him. This is such a visual story and it lightens all things at the moment!

At that same conference, I tried an experiment. Something I had done in the presence of dear friends and even my husband—and I had watched them enjoy a moment ... at my expense! I suggested that we all have loved ones, and we all have that *special look* we give our husbands when we would like a little more *loving* ... I then gave them permission to laugh, as I was going to demonstrate the look I can only give to my husband because of the muscles in my face reacting differently than before ... so they all watched me intently as I *lovingly looked their way*...my face contorts into a clown-like image ... and they break out in a boisterous laughter! Interesting, inside I feel like the look is what I always had for Hank ... but folk's reaction, including Hank's, tells me that that just isn't so!

Spending time with friends who have known me with this affliction since the beginning, is such a blessing ... they tell me I am looking better all the time, make me want to extend my horizons and really are gifts from my Heavenly Father. They are here in my life for a reason. It took me some time to just *be myself* with anyone ... but now it is OK, I no longer feel the need to explain, "I have Bell's Palsy, excuse my appearance," which I did almost every time I met someone new, whether it was a clerk, a new church member, or someone on the street, who just couldn't resist staring.

OCTOBER, 2013

It was Sunday, and we went to church as is our custom. Hank dropped me off at the main entrance, where he and I served for 10 years as greeters. I was greeted by a person new to me that I did not recognize since the serving folks have changed since our time, walked in and noticed a greeter who was still *serving* inside greeting. I went over to him and touched his arm, said "hello" and said how good it was to see him again. The difference being that he has always been serving from his wheelchair, unable to move anything but his eyes. What his days must be like … I had never thought of his *plight* before, just always gave him a "hello" and a pleasant word. Now I pray for him! He's making a difference in the world, in his own way!

An usher, who always has a nice, comforting word for me, asked how it was going and told me I was looking so much better. I told him everything seems to be as good as it seems to be going to get, but I still struggle with the left side of my mouth not wanting to move, when I'm talking, making me talk out of one side of my mouth … and eating is still a challenge. Smiling, he says that the "look" isn't bad, and it's perhaps meant to be "my signature"!

When one is afflicted with Bell's Palsy it is as though you have been singled out and you find yourself alone in a situation that no one can understand unless they too have had the disease. My eye doctor, Dr. Gary Morgan, shared that he had experienced having Bell's Palsy four times in his life so far. I cannot imagine going through all this that many times! Because he does not have a fair complexion, you really cannot see the droop in that one eye … or know that the left side of his face still does not feel "normal." So, I wonder, is this the one time I will have the disease, or will it return? Like a thief in the night, it would be just as devastating as the first time.

CHAPTER 11

THE GARAGE SALE EXPERIENCE

WHAT IS THE definition of a "garage sale"? Well, it is where one displays all their extra stuff to sell to others who might just need what you no longer need. One dreams of a <u>really great sale</u> and so you work really hard to that end. Sorting, discarding things no one will want ... even though your first thought is ... I just can't part with this! It's watching folks look carefully or not so carefully through your *things*, and keep walking on or just buying a trivial item or two ... when you are thinking, why wouldn't anyone just bring a truck (or a padded van so not to hurt anything) and buy it all? It just doesn't work that way, at least it didn't for us.

For three months we really worked to put together a garage sale. Our basement is full of stuff! Not what we need or even want ... but what we have collected and just couldn't let go. When I think of it all ... it has been like a disease in itself. You know better than to keep everything and pile it all up. After all, I have had 70 years to do that and so has Hank. There are so many people in the world without any stuff ... and here we are sitting on top of a mountain of stuff. So we diligently made the decision that this was not going to be who we are anymore!

Weeding out boxes of things to determine what goes in the garage sale and what goes to the needy or what just gets tossed out is a full time job and takes guts! No one wants to help you or offers to do it for you … so many of your family or friends are busy with their lives … so why would they want to do something that you yourself are dreading? Before Bell's, I would think about this that should be done, and then always, always just forget to start! Accidently on purpose!

So it all began, this urge to get started, at church—with an exercise our minister asked us all to do one Sunday morning. We were all given a piece of paper and a pen as we walked into church and then he asked us to write down something we needed to be prayed for and give that piece of paper to a perfect stranger before we left that day. So I did that … the idea was that the stranger was to pray for you every day … and we were to see how that worked in our lives!

The prayer I asked for was for me to be strong enough and willing to start cleaning out the basement of stuff for a garage sale. I didn't think any more about this till after a week or so when I realized that I had actually been working every day with an energy in me that was like a locomotive chugging along just pushing through box after box of stuff, making decisions that I never could before as to the fate of each individual item! Could this be my prayer being answered? This went on for over a week … my getting up early, downstairs working … Hank helping get the stuff up and out … both of us falling into bed every night exhausted.

Then one day, I woke with no enthusiasm to keep going! I smiled, realizing that that prayer person had done his or her job for a week praying for me … so now I prayed that same prayer, wanting that energy and enthusiasm back so that we could continue!

It still was a lot of hard work just for us to put the items in some sort of order in our driveway, priced and ready. Part of the battle was I just believed that I would get the strength again and, sure enough, it happened a few days later. I found myself almost running around doing what needed to be done and putting together boxes of things priced out for the sale. It was a start!

However, the success of those two short days, was not the sale of what was offered but the people who I had never met. They showed lot of interest in who we are and how our lives sort of corresponded with their own. I lost myself in their stories and forgot about the Palsy look.

A lady stopped at the end of our driveway, walked toward me and I realized that she must have Bell's Palsy as well, her face being so distorted. She looked and smiled as only she could and I found myself saying to her, "excuse me I just wanted to say that I too have the affliction you have." Thinking this would be some sort of a bond that would establish between two strangers, suffering with all the stigmas that are associated with this "look." Then she smiled and said, "No, I don't have Bell's, this look was caused in surgery years ago, when a doctor was doing something near my eye and cut a nerve." Oh my, I felt ridiculous having said what I said to her ... and thought how she must feel ...

Because of this particular incident, I have become more aware, more sensitive and more compassionate to others with different afflictions or ability levels.

CHAPTER 12

ATTITUDE

RECENTLY I HEARD of a young man, Zach Hodskins, who was born without the lower half of one arm. His family lives in Alpharetta, GA, where he grew up not feeling handicapped but determined to be the best that he could be. His accomplishments only prove that the human spirit is capable of awesome, seemingly impossible feats. At 17 he has been offered a spot on the University of Florida's elite Division 1 basketball program. There have been other athletes before him who played sports with similar handicaps ... so we know that there are challenges that are faced and conquered, but we never believe that we ourselves will have to face such things.

Each day has been a challenge. However, now I do not find myself thinking each moment of my affliction as I did early on. My mind is full of other things. How can we make our days simpler now and focus on life's simpler avenues?

A close friend of mine recently shared a piece written by Charles Swindoll, and I quote ...

ATTITUDE

"The longer I live, the more I realize the impact of attitude on my life. Attitude to me is more important than facts. It is more important than the past, than education, than money, than circumstances, than failures, than successes, than what other people think or say or do. It is more important than appearance, giftedness or skill. It will make or break a company ... a church ... a home. *The remarkable thing is we have a choice everyday regarding the attitude we will embrace for that day.* We cannot change our past ... we cannot change the fact that people will act in a certain way. We cannot change the inevitable. The only thing we can do is play on the string we have, and that is our attitude ... *I am convinced that life is 10% what happens to me and 90% how I react to it.* And so it is with us ... we are in charge of our attitudes."

I keep this where I can read it every morning. Surely you can wake in the morning and have an attitude of not being worth anything ... because everything is a struggle ... just getting ready for the day, coping with those around you and just daily life in general. You could also *choose* to wake up with a smile, an attitude of hope for what the day will bring and what you can do to make someone else feel or have that same joyful attitude.

I now wake up with thoughts of how the day might go. I have a list in my head of what needs to be done. First I say to myself, "I feel great," and pray (the **ACTS** prayer) <u>a</u>cknowledging God, <u>c</u>onfessing my sins of yesterday, <u>thanking</u> him for all He's provided and <u>surrendering</u> myself to Him.

FEBRUARY, 2014

It is now the middle of February, 2014, and I still have Bell's Palsy. I continue to work with my speech. My left eye wants to close now, the nerves seem not to do as they once did, but with stretching, by pulling the skin away from the eye, and with a conscious effort to open my eye wider I can assume a better appearance.

However I am working with my doctor who believes there is hope and I am now talking better. I notice that my posture affects my face a lot. If I am slouching, my face droops, if I hold myself in the correct posture, my face softens.

We learn lessons from the experiences we live through. Whether we choose to rethink or redo how we live is our choice. If we go forward without considering those lessons, then we do not grow, but fall back into our old life pattern.

June 8, 2014 – today, there is so much to be thankful for and even though I still have issues with my Palsy, I feel blessed in knowing that the lessons I've learned just might give someone else Hope!!

One is never the same after Bell's, but one can go on living each day with a renewed sense of purpose. For me it has been to show more love and to be more aware of my Father's influence in my life by making sure I spend those 15 minutes a day reading His word (the Bible), then waiting for His teaching hand to show me how to use His lesson in my day.

CHAPTER 13

OTHER'S VIEW

Remembering that laughter is the greatest healer and is the one thing free to us that we can use in helping others, I can still make children laugh with funny looks that I could not do before Bell's. Our youngest grandson sat on my lap, and explored my feature before asking if it hurt, what happened and laughed when I made a funny face at him. From that time on, he would tell me whether or not he saw improvements.

Children have such an innocence that they can relate to matters in such a way that is refreshing and sometimes raw! Looking into my face with wide-eyed honesty, a neighbor's grandchild tells me that my lower lip is larger than it used to be and that she hopes it gets better soon—whereas an adult would probably say nothing about the appearance, so as not to embarrass me

We recently participated in a "5K Color Run" in Louisville, KY. It was a run for charity, and you were to be splattered along the way with colored powder that turned into a paint, changing your clothes and skin into multi-colored splotches!

Because of the weight we both had lost and our daily "training," we were able to complete the run. However, when pictures were taken, afterwards I looked at my images standing in the midst of our team members and could not recognize my face. It was so distorted and looked almost like that first image I had seen in the mirror!

No one said anything at the time, but I know they must have been puzzled as I would have been—if I had known!

The next day, my face seemed to redo by itself and was back to my "normal" look as it is today. What caused that change? I don't know. Since then, I've learned that I can expect days when I am not truly looking like _I would like_ and this is something that I have accepted.

I have learned that certain situations cause a direct reaction to how I look. When I have deprived myself of a 7-8 hour sleep, whether it be from traveling or worrying, I can expect the left side of my face to look smashed and wrinkly. Any cold draft is devastating to the left side of my face as it causes swelling in addition to my left eye appearing smaller and squinty. Massaging and stretching my skin eventually helps to soften the look and feel.

When cold air is blowing directly on the left side of my face, it causes my face to swell. If I have slept hard on my left side and my face has been buried into the pillow, stretching of the left side of my mouth when I get up is necessary for my speech not to be slurred, as my tongue then seems to be off-center. Then once the stretching happens, the tongue feels normal again.

I have been sustained by the support and encouragement from loving friends and family members, even when I felt I had entered my darkest hour. There were many times I felt the need to talk about what was going on in that moment, whether it be my emotional roller coaster or the "look" I was dealing with that particular day. The shock of seeing me was sometimes overwhelming for those close … and their reaction, often bringing them to tears, was difficult for me to witness. Remember, on the inside, I still felt like my old self. Even though there was discomfort, there was nothing that should be abnormal to others. It was then that I understood just how my looks really affected others.

My husband Hank, in the beginning, diligently taped my left eye shut every night before bed, so that my eye would not completely dry up. He has always wished he could have traded places with me and had been the one stricken with this Palsy. In his mind, a woman's facial appearance is extremely important, but not as much for a man. It's been a painful time for him as well, but he has been my rock. I have been so blessed that his strength held me together throughout this time.

Nancy and Gordie, neighbors we've been close to for many years, have invited us to their house for a meal many times … and they've acted as though nothing had changed, giving me the strength I needed to face others. Nancy teared up the first time she saw me and then her caring questions and insights helped me know what I would say later to those inquiring about my *status*.

CHAPTER 14

CONCLUSIONS

I REMEMBER SKYPING with friends from Florida immediately after I had been diagnosed. They were very supportive. I had said that my looks were devastating to me and I was having a hard time dealing with it all. Our friend Joseph looked at me and just said, "Kay, it doesn't matter, you are beautiful on the inside." That one phrase, has been my *lifeline* and has pulled me through some depressing moments.

Joseph is no longer with us, as he passed due to an inoperable tumor that he had lived with for many years. Yet, his life was full of love and encouragement for others. Sally, his life partner, shared that as soon as they had turned off the Skype, Joseph broke down in tears.

But through all of this I have learned that we can *conquer* anything in this life, if we remember "We are more than conquerors through Him who loved us." (Romans 8:37)

APRIL, 2015

The past two winters have been very harsh in the Chicagoland area. I spent every outing wrapped up in a very warm scarf that was a gift from a friend of mine on my birthday. It is made of soft yarn, and has no beginning and no end, since it is made in a circular fashion. The scarf was designed to wrap around your neck a couple of times, a fashionable warm attire. I wrapped it around my neck, then around my head, covering the left side of my face so that the cold frigid air could not reach my skin. I would put a soft knitted, stretchy hat on top of this to keep everything in place. There were times when I was in the passenger side of our van, when we would pull up to another car at a stop light and I would find the driver of the other car looking at me with questioning eyes, as though I was some type of threat to him/her. With that I would pull back my head covering, showing my light-colored hair and that person would actually show me a smile of relief as we proceeded on our separate ways.

When it is really cold outside, I press a warm wash cloth to the left side of my face before going to bed. This procedure relaxes the muscles in my face, allowing me to fall asleep without the sense of stiffness on the left side. I also learned that sleeping on my back was a way to insure I would not sleep on the left side of my face. This habit also helped me to sit straighter and walk straighter during my waking hours.

I have been on the journey of trying to get this story out to those who have been struggling with the same issues I have encountered and find it frustrating that I've drawn a blank everywhere I turned in accomplishing this effort. How about publishing this as a book? This sounded easy enough, but there were obstacles in my way. First, looking for a publisher, one who would do the book justice (in my eyes). I found, looking on the internet, there are a lot of reputable publishing companies out there willing to work wonders, for a fee. After conversations and finally almost giving up, I discovered an e-book opportunity, where the book might be self-published online and reach so many more readers than I ever could have imagined.

I have included some pictures to show the journey I've been on.

Before Bell's Palsy

With Bell's Palsy, July, 2012

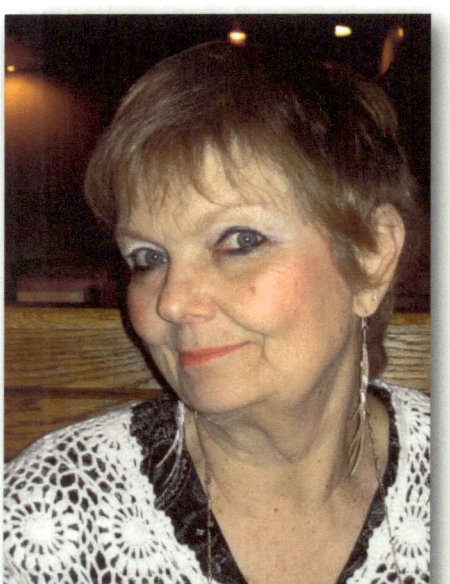

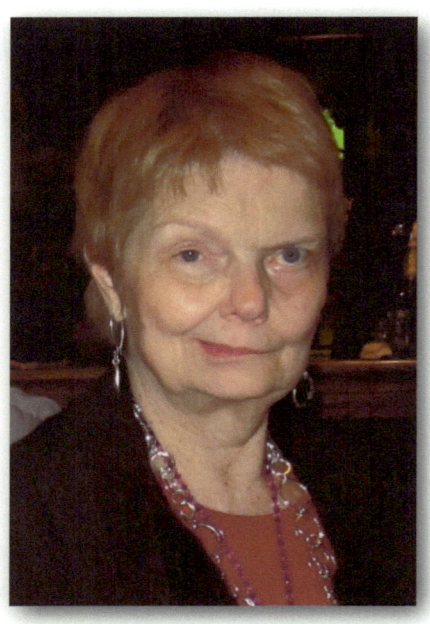

OCTOBER 2012

This is what the mirror showed me!

Who was I…..?

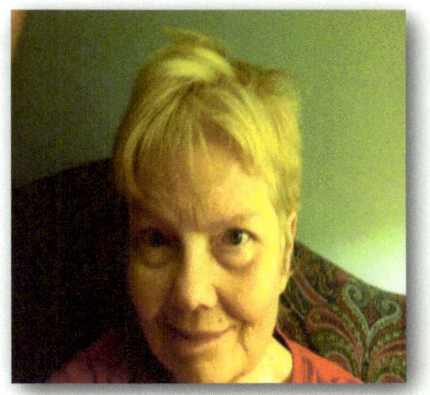

Every day I changed…

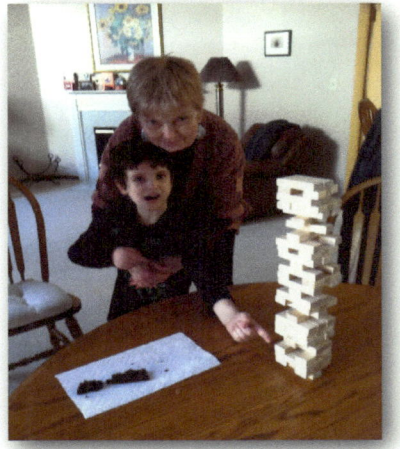

Here with EJ, our youngest grandson, my biggest fan …

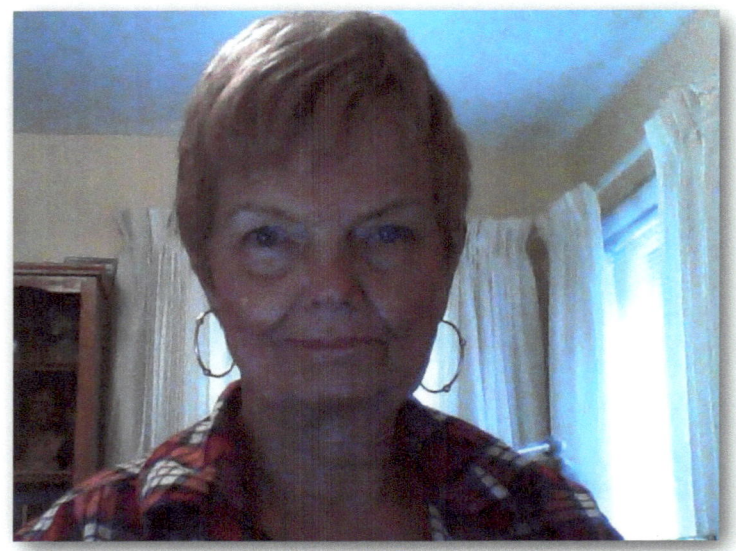

And today ... by the Grace of God ... still with issues of speech and eating, but full of hope and Blessings!

ACKNOWLEDGEMENTS

THE CHALLENGE I was given by Rev. Harvey Carey of Detroit, Michigan, to write my story, was the beginning impetus for this writing.

Reading a book by our minister Bill Hybels, *"simplify"*, also encouraged me to do what I've always wanted to do but felt I had no time to do. So now I am looking forward to my next book! Thank you.

Without a chance meeting on a flight to Florida, when I met a person, Daniel Bauer from Chicago, who shared his excitement in what he was learning about writing an e-book, I would have never thought it possible that I could publish this book I was writing, due to the cost involved in publishing a hardback copy.

Hank Balgemann, my husband and my friend. His enthusiasm has been my constant inspiration. He did the first editing of the manuscript and designed the book cover. Thank you, Hank.

Those who read my first version, suggested edits and encouraged me to share with others … thank you all so very much. I also wish to thank Al Bagdonas from South Carolina, for his final editing and proofreading.

To find out more about this journey or about my future plans for e-books, please contact me at my email address: looked.in.mirror@gmail.com. A web page is being developed now.

I would appreciate it if you would respect my desire for you not to share or distribute the e-book to anyone else without my permission.

Thank you!

Kay

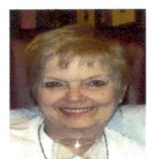

ABOUT THE AUTHOR

KAY BALGEMANN, 72 years young, is a wife, mother, grandmother and previous owner of a food business. Throughout her life, she has gained first-hand knowledge of dealings with palsy disorders. Her first encounter occurred when she gave birth to her son, BJ Dugan, who had Cerebral Palsy from birth.

BJ was born with a cleft palate, slight Cerebral Palsy, making it difficult for him to walk, talk or sit up. At his two-month exam, Kay insisted on a second opinion wanting to determine why BJ would not look at toys, turn himself over or reach for his mom or dad. No longer taking the doctor's assurance that boys are usually slow, Kay and her husband took BJ to see the head neurologist at Loyola University, Dr. Vuckovich, in Chicago, who took BJ on as a patient.

It was soon discovered that he could neither hear nor see. After getting glasses for his eyes to see and tubes in his ears so he could hear, we were all looking forward to new beginnings. With testing and training he learned sign language, and to scoot instead of crawling. Braces were to be fitted for his legs as he was growing stronger and he was expected to begin to walk. Then his kidneys stopped growing when he was almost 5 years of age.

The family then had almost a year caring for him, his older sister Cheryl, being his greatest cheerleader. He passed and now Easter Baskets are donated to Lurie's Children Hospital in Chicago every year in BJ's memory.

Kay lives with her husband, Henry Balgemann, Sr. in Villa Park, IL. Kay's daughter, Cheryl Gribbens and her husband Emmett and son Emmett (EJ) live in Gurnee, IL.; stepdaughter Wendy Zobel lives with her husband Fred in Wheaton, IL; stepson, Robert Balgemann and wife Angie live in the Nashville, Tennessee area, along with their children Raeanne Balgemann, Baylee Balgemann and Robert Balgemann. Henry Balgemann, Jr. lives in AZ.

This has been Kay's first attempt at writing, and she plans to continue writing both on this true life topic and on fictional stories, close to her heart.